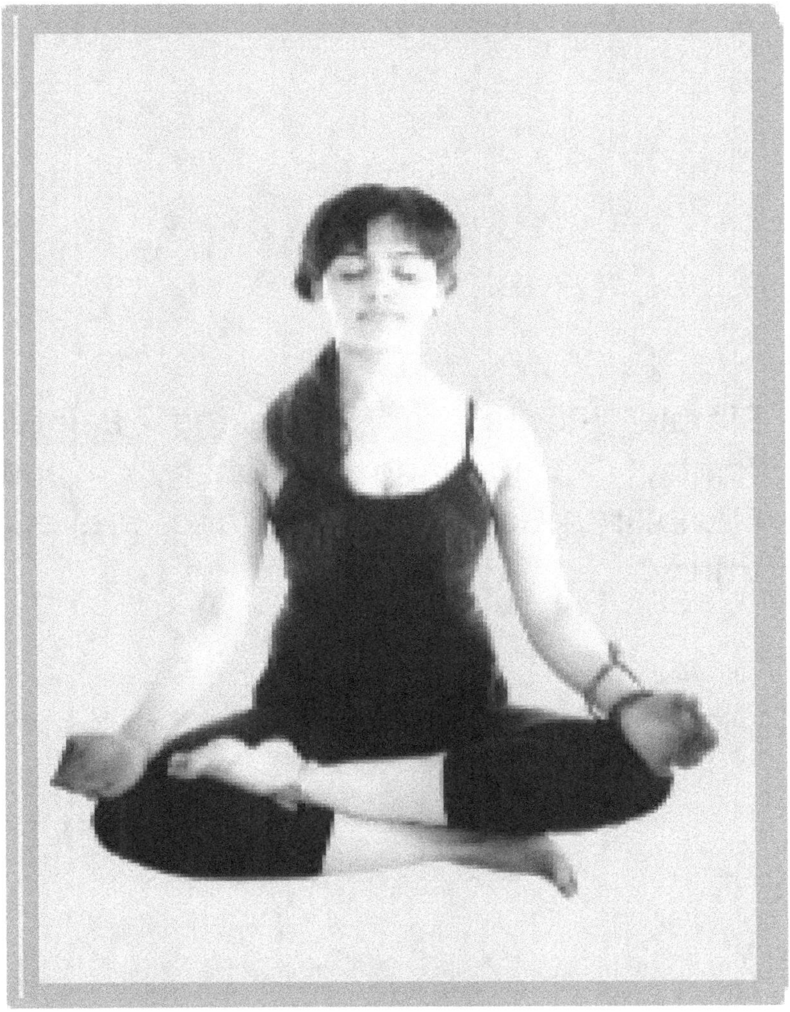

40 YOGIC EXERCISES FOR ARTHRITIS

Simple Poses for Relieving Painful Joints, Improving Mobility and Flexibility, Build Muscles, and Prevent Injury.

PAUL KELVIN

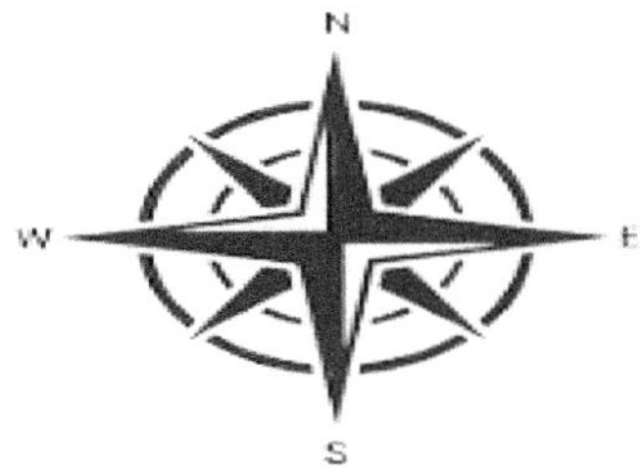

TABLE OF CONTENTS

INTRODUCTION

Pain from arthritis can take away the pleasure of daily tasks, leaving you feeling constrained and irritated. However, what if there was a drug-free, all-natural method to reduce your discomfort, increase your range of motion, and take back control of your body?

40 Yogic Exercises for Arthritis is the key to utilizing yoga's therapeutic benefits for controlling your arthritis pain.

Anyone who wants to feel better and move more easily, regardless of age or skill level, will benefit from this thorough approach.

Anyone who is most likely struggling with arthritis this book is for you. Arthritis may be an unwelcome but continuous friend.

It can cause persistent pains that make everyday activity become intimidating or tight joints that make getting out of bed in the mornings difficult.

Instead of seeing yoga as a fad in the fitness world, see it as a lifesaver a simple, non-threatening means of taking back control of my physical and mental well-being. It is important to know that this book is designed with you in mind.

One may ask, "Why yoga?" The solution is straightforward yet profound: yoga provides an all-encompassing method of relieving pain associated with arthritis.

To encourage internal healing, it's not only about stretching or working out physically; it's also about establishing a connection between your body, mind, and soul. Yoga fosters a sense of peace and well-being while assisting with flexibility, strength, and balance.

This book contains 40 well-chosen yoga poses created especially for people with arthritis. Every exercise is explained in detail, with easy-to-follow directions and illustrations to make sure you can do it. These exercises, which vary from easy stretches to more strenuous positions, are all designed to increase mobility and reduce discomfort.

The personal touch is what makes this book unique. This is a handbook written by someone who genuinely knows what you're going through, not simply a list of exercises.

I added guidance on listening to your body, suggestions for adapting each posture to fit your requirements, and motivational words to keep you going. Every chapter is designed to assist you on your path to pain reduction by offering ideas and experiences in a conversational style.

Within this book, you will find out:

- An explanation of arthritis in simple terms, along with how yoga may be your most effective ally in controlling it.

- Easy breathing techniques called pranayama might help you feel better overall and less pained.
- 40 secure and beneficial yoga poses created especially to address frequent arthritis-affected locations.
- Well-planned poses for your back, hips, knees, ankles, feet, shoulders, and hands.
- yoga poses are created especially to reduce morning stiffness, enhance the quality of your sleep, and broaden your range of motion.
- Modifications and lifestyle advice to help you easily include yoga into your everyday schedule.

This book provides a comprehensive approach to arthritis management, beyond merely exercises. Discover how to develop a long-lasting yoga practice and your general well-being.

Imagine experiencing pain-free mornings, effortless movement, and restored body confidence.

40 Yoga Asanas for Arthritis A path to a better, happier version of yourself is marked by painLeave it now, don't delay. Begin your path to a life free of pain right now!

CHAPTER 1: UNDERSTANDING ARTHRITIS AND HOW YOGIC EXERCISES CAN BE USED TO MANAGE ARTHRITIS

Swelling and pain in one or more joints are symptoms of arthritis. The primary signs and symptoms of arthritis are stiffness and pain in the joints, which usually get worse with age. The two most prevalent forms of arthritis are rheumatoid arthritis and osteoarthritis.

The firm, slick cartilage that covers the ends of bones where they meet to create a joint breaks away due to osteoarthritis. In rheumatoid arthritis, the illness, the immune system targets the joints, starting with the joint lining.

Gout can result from uric acid crystals, which occur when there is an excess of uric acid in the blood. Other forms of arthritis can be brought on by infections or underlying medical conditions like lupus or psoriasis.

The kind of arthritis determines the different treatments. Improving quality of life and reducing symptoms are the major objectives of arthritis therapy.

TYPES OF ARTHRITIS PAIN:

The different arthritis include:

Axial spondyloarthritis: this is another name for ankylosing spondylitis, is an inflammatory condition that can eventually lead to the fusion of certain vertebrae, or spine bones. This fusion might cause a slumped posture and reduce the spine's flexibility.

It might be harder to breathe deeply if the ribs are affected.

Gout Arthritis: Anyone can develop gout, a common and complex form of arthritis that is characterized by sudden, severe attacks of discomfort, redness, swelling, and pain in one or more joints, most commonly the big toe. Gout attacks can happen suddenly, often waking you up in the middle of the night with the feeling that your big toe is on fire. The affected joint is hot, swollen, and so tender that even the weight of the bedsheet may seem unbearable around it.

Juvenile idiopathic arthritis: Children under the age of sixteen most commonly suffer from juvenile idiopathic arthritis, formerly known as juvenile rheumatoid arthritis.

 An ongoing source of joint discomfort, swelling, and stiffness is juvenile idiopathic arthritis.

For a few months, for a few years, or even years, some children may have symptoms.
Serious side effects, such as growth issues, joint damage, and inflammation in the eyes, can result in some forms of juvenile idiopathic arthritis. Managing discomfort and inflammation, enhancing

performance, and averting harm are the main goals of treatment.

Osteoarthritis: Millions of people worldwide suffer from osteoarthritis, the most prevalent kind of arthritis. It happens as the cartilage that cushions both ends of the bones ages and becomes less effective.

While osteoarthritis may harm any joint, it most frequently affects the hands, knees, hips, and spine.

Although joint damage cannot be undone, osteoarthritis symptoms are typically manageable.

Remaining physically active, keeping a healthy weight, and undergoing certain therapies may assist in reducing discomfort and enhancing joint function while also slowing the disease's progression.

Septic arthritis: An excruciating pain in the joints known as "septic arthritis" may be caused by bacteria that enter your circulation from another area of your body. Additionally, penetrating injuries (such as animal bites or traumas) that allow bacteria to enter the joint directly might cause septic arthritis.

Septic arthritis is more common in older persons and infants. It can also strike people with prosthetic joints. Septic arthritis primarily affects the knees, although it can also affect the hips, shoulders, and other joints. Treatment must begin as soon as possible since the infection has the potential to swiftly and severely harm the joint's bone and cartilage.

During surgery or as part of treatment, the joint is drained using a needle. Antibiotics are typically required as well.

Psoriatic arthritis: This is a kind of arthritis that individuals with psoriasis (a skin condition characterized by red skin areas covered in silvery scales) experience. Before being diagnosed with psoriatic arthritis, the majority of patients first acquire psoriasis. However, for some, the joint issues start concurrently with or before the skin patches do.

The primary indicators and symptoms of psoriatic arthritis include joint pain, stiffness, and edema. They can range in severity from moderate to severe and affect any area of the body, including your fingers and spine. Periods of remission can alternate with flare-ups of the illness in both psoriasis and psoriatic arthritis.

It is not possible to treat psoriatic arthritis. The goals of treatment are to manage symptoms and avoid joint deterioration. Psoriatic arthritis can be quite debilitating if left untreated.

Rheumatoid arthritis: This kind of arthritis is an inflammatory disease that can affect more than just the joints the Skin, eyes, lungs, heart, and blood vessels are just a few of the systems in the body that might sustain harm from the illness in certain individuals.

Rheumatoid arthritis is an autoimmune disease that happens when your immune system unintentionally targets the tissues in your own body. It affects the lining of your joints, generating discomfort and swelling that may eventually contribute to bone erosion and joint deformity, unlike the wear-and-tear deterioration of osteoarthritis.

Rheumatoid arthritis-related inflammation is what causes harm to other bodily components as well. Even though there are now many more treatment choices available due to new drugs, severe rheumatoid arthritis can still cause physical limitations.

Thumb arthritis: This is frequently associated with ageing and arises from the wear and tear of cartilage from both ends of the joint bones that make up the carpometacarpal (CMC) joint, which is located at the base of your thumb.

Simple actions like opening jars and turning doorknobs can become challenging due to the acute discomfort, swelling, and reduced strength and range of motion caused by thumb arthritis. Splints and medicines are typically used in conjunction with treatment. One may need surgery for severe thumb arthritis.

Reactive arthritis: This is characterized by joint pain and swelling that is brought on by an infection in another bodily area, usually the urinary system, genitalia, or intestines.

Usually, this ailment affects the feet, ankles, and knees. Inflammation can also impact the skin, eyes, and urethra, the tube that exits the body with pee. Reiter's syndrome was the previous term used to describe reactive arthritis. Rarely can reactive arthritis occur.

Most patients experience intermittent indications and symptoms that go away after a year.

THE COMMON SYMPTOMS OF ARTHRITIS:

The joints are the primary site of arthritis indications and symptoms. The symptoms and indications of arthritis can vary depending on the kind and may involve the following:

- Pain in the joints.
- Restricted range of movement, or stiffness in a joint's range of motion.
- Oedema (an inflammation).
- Discoloration of the skin.
- hypersensitivity to touch or discomfort around a joint.
- A sensation of warmth or heat close to your joints.

The type of arthritis you have and the joints it affects determine where you feel symptoms. Flares, also known as flare-ups, are periodic waves of symptoms caused by some kinds of arthritis. Others cause constant pain or stiffness in your joints, especially after physical activity.

Note: if you are feeling the symptoms above ensure that you visit the doctor or a health care provider for a proper body examination.

CAUSES OF ARTHRITIS

Depending on the kind, many things could cause arthritis:

- Age-related osteoarthritis develops naturally as a result of lifelong joint use that wears down the cartilage that cushions the joint.
- Hyperuricemia, or high blood uric acid, increases the risk of developing gout.
- Rheumatoid arthritis is one type of arthritis that can result from your immune system accidentally injuring your joints.

- Arthritis can be caused by certain viral infections, such as COVID-19.
- Arthritis can occasionally occur without a cause or trigger. Physicians refer to the condition as idiopathic arthritis.

What are the risk factors?

Although anybody can have arthritis, several things might increase your risk, such as:

- Use of tobacco products: Using tobacco products, including smoking, raises your risk.
- **Family history:** Individuals are more prone to arthritis if they have biological family members who already have it.
- **Activity level:** If you don't engage in regular physical activity, you may be at higher risk of developing arthritis.
- **Medical conditions:** The likelihood of developing arthritis is

increased if you have any autoimmune disorders, are obese, or have any other condition that affects your joints.

- Gender: Although gout, another kind of arthritis, is primarily experienced by males, women are more likely than men to get rheumatoid arthritis.
- **Prior arthritic injury**: Arthritis is more likely to develop in a joint that a person has hurt, maybe during sports.
- **Being overweight**. Stress on joints, especially the knees, hips, and spine, results from being overweight. An increased risk of arthritis development exists in obese individuals.

TREATMENT AND MANAGEMENT OF ARTHRITIS:

Although there isn't a cure for arthritis, your doctor can help you identify therapies to help manage your symptoms. The cause of your arthritis, the kind you have, and the joints it affects will determine the treatments you require.

Among the most popular therapies for arthritis are:

- NSAIDs and acetaminophen are examples of over-the-counter (OTC) anti-inflammatory medications.
- Corticosteroids are anti-inflammatory prescription drugs, such as cortisone shots.
- If you have psoriatic or rheumatoid arthritis, you should take disease-modifying antirheumatic medications (DMARDs).
- Physical therapy such as exercises can be helpful to some kind of arthritis. Exercises such as yoga can strengthen the muscles that surround joints and increase the range of motion. Braces or splints

could be necessary in some situations.

- Surgery (typically reserved for cases in which nonsurgical measures fail to alleviate symptoms).

PREVENTION:

Arthritis is not always preventable. Age and family history are two examples of things that are beyond your control.

But as you age, a few good practices might help lower your chance of experiencing joint discomfort. The various ways to prevent arthritis include:

- Always eat food that contains omega-3 fatty acids. According to research omega 3s reduces the RA activity in the joint. The food that consists of omega-3 fatty acids are; sardine, salmon, trout, mackerel, fortified eggs, soya beverage nuts and seeds such as walnuts, chia seeds, flaxseeds, and many more.

Note: omega-3 acids supplements are also available in different doses.

- Keeping a modest weight might help reduce arthritis discomfort. In America, around 23% of overweight individuals and 31% of obese individuals have been diagnosed with arthritis. For those with knee OA, losing one pound of weight can relieve four pounds of strain on the knees. Compared to decreasing 5% of body weight, dropping 10% to 20% of beginning body weight can significantly improve function, quality of life, and discomfort.
- Give up smoking: It might be challenging to break the habit.

However, giving up smoking helps prevent arthritis in addition to lowering the risk of lung and heart problems.

- Keep an eye on your blood sugar: Diabetes and arthritis have a reciprocal association. The Centers for Disease Control and Prevention (CDC) report that arthritis affects 47% of adult Americans with diabetes (Trusted Source). The chance of having diabetes is 61% greater in people with arthritis.
- Increase your ergonomics: It is possible to avoid further strain and discomfort on already painful joints by arranging your house and office more ergonomically. Assume enough support for your arms, legs, and back if you must sit for extended amounts of time at work.
- Guard your joints: Future joint issues may arise from knee bending, climbing, kneeling, hard lifting, and squatting. Joints might be particularly strained by lifting.

Additional risk factors for osteoarthritis are standing and vibration exposure.

Several of the occupations that are most prone to cause joint issues

- engage in routine exercise: Engaging in Exercise strengthens the muscles surrounding your joints and relieves the strain that comes with carrying extra weight. They are stabilized and may be shielded from damage by this.

If you engage in different yogic exercises at least five days a week, it will improve your overall fitness help to shade some of the weight in your joints, and make you feel lighter.

However, in the remaining chapters of this book, you will practice various yogic exercises that will help to strengthen the entire joints and improve your overall fitness.

BENEFITS OF YOGA FOR ARTHRITIS:

According to research, studies have shown in the past years that Yoga's meditative features make it a safe and effective technique to promote physical activity, and it also provides significant psychological advantages. Yoga can help with balance, respiratory endurance, flexibility, muscle strength, and strength, much as other types of exercise.

Yoga is linked to less physical aches and pains as well as more vitality.

Lastly, studies have shown that yoga improves psychological stress, anxiety, and sadness.

In conclusion, there are many different physical and psychological advantages linked to yoga, which may be particularly beneficial for those who are coping with a chronic condition.

whenever you start feeling the symptoms of arthritis please ensure you see a doctor or rheumatologist before you start any treatment or exercise for arthritis also you must consult your if you have an injury before you participate in any of this exercise routine.

SAFETY MEASURES FOR YOGIC POSES FOR ARTHRITIS:

For you to get started with any of the yoga poses for arthritis, you must take the following measures.

Speak with your physician: This is essential to make sure yoga is safe for the particular kind and degree of arthritis you have. Talk about any restrictions or changes you might require.

Locate a certified yoga instructor: Seek out a yoga instructor who has received certification in yoga for arthritis or who has expertise teaching people with the condition.

Pay attention to your body: Pain is an indication to quit! Don't push yourself past what seems comfortable. Adjust your positions or take a break as required.

It's crucial to warm up: Your joints become ready for activity with gentle exercises like arm circles, neck rolls, and short stretches.

Set up your surroundings: Locate a peaceful, cosy area with a non-slip yoga mat. Props like straps, bolsters, and blocks can be used to adjust and provide additional support.

Put on comfortable attire: Clothing that fits loosely permits free movement.

WHEN ENGAGING IN YOGA:

Yoga stresses breathing and synchronized movement, so pay attention to your breath.

Breathe in during contraction and out during expansion.

Preserve correct alignment: To prevent joint tension, a trained teacher may assist in making sure that you are using the right form.

Proceed carefully and slowly: Prioritize movement quality over intensity or speed.

Adjust poses: Don't be afraid to change positions to meet your demands. If a posture is uncomfortable, modify your arm and leg positions or utilize props for support.

Remain hydrated: Before, during, and after your practice, make sure you consume lots of water.

Properly cool down: Your body may return to a resting state with the aid of gentle stretches and relaxation positions like Child's Pose.

Extra Advice:

- Talk to your instructor: Tell them you have arthritis and any associated limitations. They can provide specific adjustments.
- Observe your body following practice: After your session, pay attention to any soreness or

stiffness that may develop. See your physician if the pain doesn't go away.
- Remain steadfast and patient: Frequent practice is more advantageous than sporadic, intensive sessions, even if it is short.

However, the materials you need to start these yoga poses are:

- Yoga mat
- Cushion
- pillow

CHAPTER 2:WARM-UPS, POSES FOR NECK SHOULDER, KNEES, ANKLE, AND HIP JOINT ARTHRITIS AND PAINS

Before participating in any kind of physical activity, especially yoga poses you must warm up your body.

 By warming up before a workout, you may protect your joints and muscles from damage and enhance your performance.

Warming up is especially crucial for those with arthritis since it helps to improve blood flow to the afflicted regions, lessen stiffness, and make movement more comfortable and easy. It doesn't have to be difficult to warm up.

It only takes a small, steady increase in exercise to fully prepare your body. The secret is to always stay inside your comfort zone, listen to your body, and take it slow while moving.

These are simple stretches you may use as part of your warm-up regimen. The purpose of these stretches is to help people with arthritis feel comfortable and in control. Never forget to take your time and breathe deeply while doing each stretch.

The warm-up for arthritis includes:

STEP UP AND OVER:

- To start this, your hands should be on the top of your hips and your feet should be shoulder-width apart.
- Slightly touch the wall in your front so you can balance.
- Step out to your right as if you are stepping over something, Once your right leg is raised to the level of your thigh, switch your weight to your left leg.
- After pausing, descend into a half-squat or squat.

- Rise to your feet take a step back to your starting position on each side, and repeat 5 times.

STEPPING UP HIGH:

- First, ensure that your feet are shoulder-width apart and also parallel to the ground.
- Then your right knee should be raised toward your chest, and take one step forward with the left leg (if necessary, steady yourself against a wall).
- To raise the knee farther, use both hands (or just one if you're using the other for balance).
- Repeat on the next side after you pause to drop the right leg.
- As you move ahead, keep "high-stepping" 5 times on each of the legs.

INSTEP TO TOE STROLL:

- Ensure that your feet are shoulder-width apart.
- Step forward a little, putting your right heel down and sliding onto your foot ball.
- Ascend vary high as you can on your toes, extending your left foot and continuing the heel-to-toe roll, and repeat 5 times for each leg.

LUNGE WITH A TWIST:

- With your feet parallel, take a big stride forward and place your right foot firmly on the floor in front of you, maintaining one hand on a wall so you can balance if necessary.
- Your body should remain straight while allowing your knee and hip to bend gradually.
- Don't allow your right knee to stretch over your toes; instead, keep it exactly over your ankle.

- Bend the left knee gently and descend it so that it is only a few inches above the ground (or as low as your flexibility will allow).
- In this position, bend your body to the right and stretch your left arm overhead (omitting the overhead reach if your shoulders are unstable).
- Go to the starting position, straighten your torso and take a stride further with your left foot. On each side, repeat 5 times. (Note: If you are having difficulty with balance, don't do this.)

STEPPING UP HIGH:

- To start this warm-up, you will have to place your toes shoulder-width apart and parallel to the ground.
- Lift your right knee in the direction of your chest while taking a step further with your left leg (if

necessary, steady yourself against a wall).

- To raise the knee farther, use both hands (or just one if you're using the other for balance).
- Repeat the next side after pausing to drop the right leg. As you move ahead, keep "high-stepping" on each leg 5 times.
- Walk from Heel to Toe. Ensure that your feet are shoulder-width apart.
- Step further a little, putting your right heel down and sliding onto the ball of your foot.
- Ascend high on your toes, extending the left foot and also continuing the heel-to-toe roll on each leg, and repeat 5 times.

ARM MOTIONS IN CIRCLES:

- First, position your feet shoulder-width apart, stretch your arms at shoulder height and your palms position down.

- Make 20 circular movements with your arms in each direction. As you gain flexibility, gradually increase the size of the circles.

ARM SWING:

- Position your arms out in front of you, parallel to the floor, with your palms positioned downward.
- Step forward and simultaneously swing the arms to the right, then bring your left arm up to your chest and point your fingers in that direction.
- Move solely at the shoulders and maintain your head and body pointing forward.
- As you take another stride, swing your arms in the next direction then repeat each side 5 times.

CIRCLES AROUND THE HIPS:

- Using a countertop as support, stand on a foot, then slowly swing the next leg out to the side in circles.

- Make 20 circles in every direction. Change your legs.
- As you gain flexibility, gently extend the size of the circles.

CHAPTER 3: YOGIC POSES FOR ARTHRITIS IN THE KNEE AND JOINT PAIN

It might be difficult to manage hip and knee arthritis, but some yoga positions can strengthen muscles, improve flexibility, and reduce pain.

Always observe your body whenever you are performing any form of exercise, if you are uncomfortable then adjust or avoid it completely. Practising yoga consistently and gently is essential to reap its advantages for arthritis.

WARRIOR I YOGA POSE:

This yoga helps to strengthen the lower back and legs, opens up the chest and hips, and enhances focus and stability.

How to do this yoga is as follows:

- Place your feet around three to four feet apart.
- Rotate your left leg gently in and your right leg 90 degrees out.

- Your right knee should be bent over your right ankle.
- Lift your arms and rotate your palms towards one another.
- After 30 to 60 seconds of holding, switch sides.

WARRIOR II YOGA POSE:

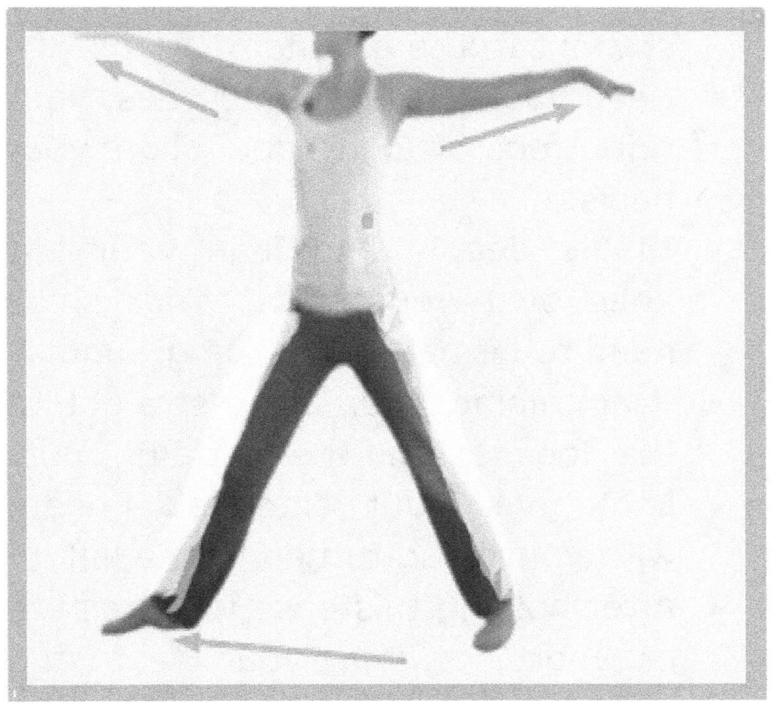

This yoga builds ankle and leg strength, groins and hips, and build endurance and concentration.

The following steps to take when doing this pose:

- Step your feet apart by approximately four feet while standing.
- Keeping your palms down, raise your arms to the front and back (not to the sides) until they are straight to the ground.
- Keep your left leg 90 degrees, your right foot straight and align your heels.
- Inhale deeply and lean your left knee over your ankle. Your shins need to be parallel to the ground.
- Maintaining your arms straight to the floor, extend them straight out.
- Look over your extended fingers with your head turned to the left.
- After holding this pose for a minute or more, switch your feet and repeat the movement on the next side.

This yoga stretches the knees, groins, and inner thighs, increases the hip joints' range of motion eases mental tension, and reduces weariness.

To do this yoga follow the instructions below:

- Stretch your legs out in front of you while you sit.
- Bring the soles of your feet together and bend your knees.
- Bend at the knees to the sides. Sit up straight and place your hands on your feet.
- Breathe deeply while holding for one to two minutes.

STAFF YOGA POSE:

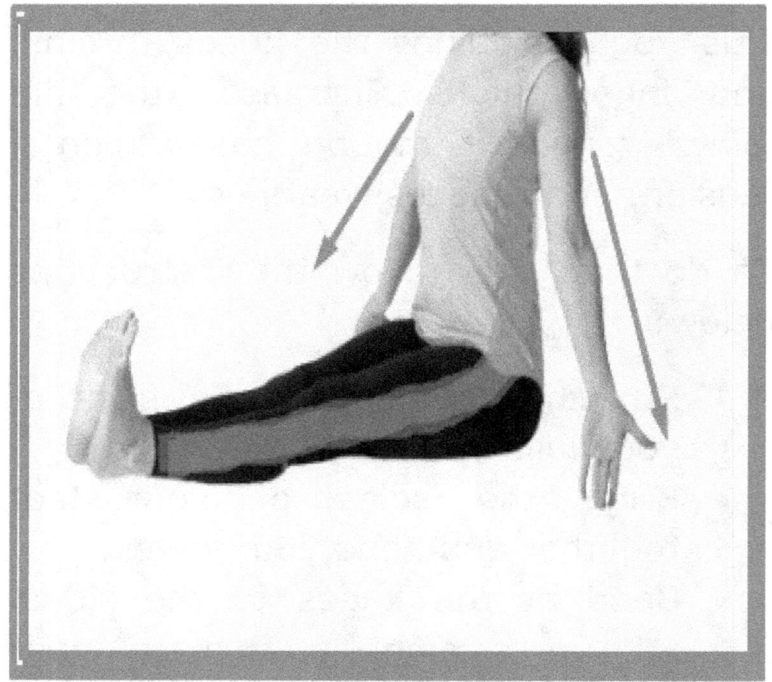

This is similar to Mountain Pose, this pose is straightforward, but the technique is key to getting the best results.

Benefits:

This yoga strengthens the neck joint, and the upper and lower back, shoulder, and hip muscles.

How to do it include:

- Sit on the floor with your legs together, and stretch them out in front of you (using a pillow or blanket to lift your pelvis can help).
- Sit against a wall to ensure proper alignment; the lower part of your back and head ought to be apart from the wall.
- Firm your thighs by pressing them down and rotating them toward each other.
- Flex your ankles while pressing out.
- Hold the pose for at least one minute.

MOUNTAIN YOGA POSE:

This yoga enhances posture, strengthens the ankles, knees, and thighs and improves stability and focus.

How to do this yoga include:

- keep your heels a bit apart and your second toes straight while standing with the sides of your big toes touching.
- Spread and raise your toes, then return them to the ground.
- You may rock side to side or back and forth to get the ideal posture.
- Having your weight distributed equally over both feet is the aim.
- Keep your spine neutral and stand tall. With your hands pointing outward, your arms should be at your sides.
- Remember to take deep breaths in and out during your one-minute hold of the position.

CHAIR YOGA POSE:

This yoga strengthens the spine, calves, and thighs stretches the upper body and chest, and improves strength and flexibility.

How to do this pose include:

- Place your feet hip-width apart as you   stand.
  Taking a breath, extend your arms over your head.
- Breathe out, bending your knees and lowering your hips to the position of a reclined chair.
- Maintain your knees behind your toes and your weight on your heels.
  While holding still for 30 seconds to 1 minute, take deep breaths.

BRIDGE YOGA POSE:

This yogic exercise strengthens the hamstrings, glutes, and back. It opens the shoulders and chest and increases the hips' and spine's flexibility.

How to do this yoga include:

- With your feet hip-width apart and your knees bent, lie on your back.
- Place your arms at your sides, palms facing down.

- As you raise your hips toward the ceiling, firmly plant your feet.
- Press your arms into the floor and interlace your fingers below your back.
- After 30 to 60 seconds of holding, drop your hips.

HAND-TO-BIG-TOE POSE IN RECLINING:

This yoga stretches the hamstrings, calves, and hips. It also reduces discomfort in the lower back and enhances alignment and flexibility.

How to do this yoga include:

- Stretch your legs out while lying on your back.
- Put a strap around your right foot and bend your right knee.
- Holding the strap with both hands, extend your right leg straight towards the sky.
- Maintain your left leg outstretched on the ground.

- After holding for one to two minutes, swap sides.

POSE WITH LEGS UP THE WALL:

This yoga relieves aching feet and minimizes inflammation and oedema. It also reduces the tension in the nervous system.

To do this yoga, follow the instructions below:

- Prop yourself up against a wall.
- Lying back, place your buttocks near the wall and swing your legs up the wall.
- Remain with your arms by your sides.
  Breathe deeply while holding for five to ten minutes.

POSE IN CAT-COW STYLE:

This yoga promotes spinal flexibility. It stretches the back, abdomen, and hips and also enhances balance and blood flow.

How to do this yoga is as follows:

- Place yourself on your hands and knees like you're on a table.
- Take a breath, raise your head and tailbone, and arch your back (Cow Pose).
- Take a breath out, arch your back, and tuck your chin in (Cat Pose).
- Breathe deeply as you alternate between Cat and Cow for another 1-2 minutes.

As part of daily practice, these yoga poses can help treat hip and knee arthritis.

Always pay attention to your body, and if a position is uncomfortable, adjust it or avoid it completely. Practising yoga consistently and gently is essential to reap its advantages for arthritis.

CHAPTER 4: YOGA POSES TO IMPROVE WRIST AND HAND ARTHRITIS PAIN

Yoga is very useful in treating wrist and hand discomfort, which is frequently brought on by arthritis, repetitive strain injuries, and other ailments.

The following yoga positions are specially meant to help strengthen, stretch, and ease wrist and hand pain:

STRETCHES FOR THE WRIST:

This yoga stretches the tendons and muscles of the forearm and wrist. It also eases stress and improves flexibility.

How to do this yoga is as follows:

- Take a comfortable seat and sit up straight.
- With your palm facing down, extend one arm in front of you.
- Stretch the top of your wrist and forearm by using your other hand to gently press your outstretched hand downward.

- Hold for ten to fifteen seconds.
- Next, extend the wrist's underside by pressing the same hand upward.
- Hold for 10-15seconds
- Conversely, repeat.

EXTEND FINGERS POSE:

This yoga increases the hands' and fingers' strength and flexibility. It eases stiffness and improves blood flow.

The guide to doing this yoga is as follows:

- Take a comfortable seat or stand. Spread your fingers as widely as you can by extending them.
- Hold on for a while.
- Form a fist and squeeze it firmly yet softly.
- Hold on for a while and repeat the steps 5–10 times.

YOGA POSE OF PRAYER:

This yoga stretches the forearm and wrist. It also enhances wrist stability and balance.

The guide to doing this yoga is as follows:

- Maintain a straight back while you sit or stand.
- Press your palms firmly together in front of your chest. Bring them together.
- Keep the same distance between your elbows and wrists.
- While holding still for 30 seconds to 1min, take deep breaths.

REVERSE PRAYER YOGA POSE:

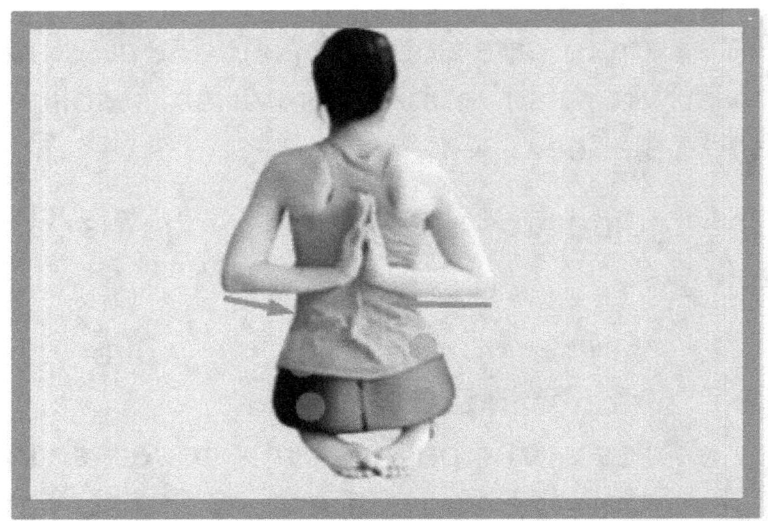

This yoga is done when you join your hands behind your back. This helps to strengthen the upper part of the body and it targets the arms and belly. It also concentrates on the wrists and shoulders. In addition to training the muscles, it helps burn fat in the arms.

The guide to doing this yoga is as follows:

- Choose a comfortable sitting position, such as Sukhasana.

Tadasana, or standing stance, is another way to perform this pose.

- Let the hands rest lightly at your sides then rest your shoulders.
- Bend your elbows and fingertips pointing down, place your hands at your back and draw in a deep breath.
- Try to contact your opposite fingertips as you exhale while rotating your hands so your fingers will be pointing at the ceiling.
- Bring the hands down to the waist side and split the palms to relax the stance.
- You can sit and rest for a few minutes with your palms resting on your thighs.

This can help to reduce shoulder stiffness by slowly rotating the shoulders in a circular motion forward as well as backward a few times. It can also release any tension in the shoulder muscles.

COW FACE YOGA POSE (ARMS ALONE):

This yoga strengthens the wrists, triceps, and shoulders, reduces stiffness, and improves flexibility.

The following are the steps to take when performing this pose:

- You can stand or comfortably sit. Bring your hand down your back and extend your right arm above while bending your elbow.
- Attempt to clench your fists together by reaching your left arm behind your back.
- Apply a strap if necessary. After 30 to 60 seconds of holding, switch sides.

DOWNWARD-FACING DOG YOGA POSE:

This yoga strengthens the arms and wrists joints, hamstrings, calves, and shoulders. Also, it enhances the alignment and balance of the entire body.

The guide to doing this yoga is as follows:

- Get on your hands and knees to begin.
- Raise your hips back and forth, extending your legs, and arranging your torso to form an inverted V.
- As you push hard into the ground with your fingers spread wide, the weight will be distributed equally across your hands.
- While holding still for 30 to 1 minute, take deep breaths.

ARMS ONLY IN EAGLE YOGA POSE:

This yoga stretches the upper back, shoulders, forearms, and wrists. Also, it eases stress and increases flexibility.

The guide to doing this yoga is as follows:

- Take a comfortable seat or stand.

- Stretch your arms out in front of you, attempting to bring your palms together while you encircle your right arm beneath your left.
- Raise your elbows to your shoulders and extend your fingers upwards.
  After 30-60 seconds of holding, switch sides.

THE MODIFIED PLANK YOGA POSE:

This yoga builds strength in the shoulders, wrists, arms, and core. Also increases the body's overall stamina and balance.

The guide to doing this yoga is as follows:

- Take a seat at a table to begin.
- Bring your body into a straight line from your head to your heels by extending your legs back and getting on your toes.
- Make fists with your hands or rest your forearms on the ground for

support rather than laying your palms flat on the ground.
- While holding still for 30 seconds to 1 minute take deep breaths.

SAVASANA (CORPORATE POSE): HAND RELAXATION:

This yoga encourages calmness and profound relaxation. It permits hands and wrists to rest and heal.

How to carry out this yoga:

- With your arms at your sides and your legs outstretched, lie flat on your back.
- Shut your eyes and unwind throughout your body.
- Let rid of any stress and concentrate on letting your hands and wrists relax.
- Hold this position for five to ten minutes while taking regular, deep breaths.

These yoga positions can help strengthen the muscles that support the wrists and hands, improve flexibility, and reduce discomfort in these regions.

Finally always practice attentively and gently, paying attention to your body and avoiding any uncomfortable motions.

CHAPTER 5: SIMPLE YOGA POSES FOR REDUCING PAIN AND IMPROVE FLEXIBILITY IN THE LOWER BACK

These yoga positions can increase flexibility, strengthen the muscles that support the lower back, and relieve discomfort associated with lower back arthritis.

Always practice attentively and gently, paying attention to your body and avoiding any uncomfortable motions.

The following are the different yoga poses for lower back arthritis:

UPINE HAMSTRINGS YOGA POSE:

This yoga strengthens the calves, hamstrings, and lower back. It reduces stress and increases mobility. it also reduces discomfort in the lower back.

The guide to doing this yoga is as follows:

- Stretch your legs out while lying on your back.
- Put a strap around your foot and bend one knee.
- Stretch your leg straight up toward the ceiling while using both hands to grip the strap.
-
  Maintain the opposite leg outstretched on the ground.
- After holding for one to two minutes, swap sides.

EXTENDED TRIANGLE YOGA POSE:

This traditional standing position may be beneficial for treating neck, sciatica, and back discomfort.

It strengthens your shoulders, chest, and legs while stretching your hips, thighs, and spine. It could also aid in anxiety and stress relief.

Targeted muscles included the medius hamstrings, quadriceps, internal oblique gluteus maximus, and latissimus dorsi.

The following are the steps to follow when performing this pose:

- Step with your feet spaced around 4 feet apart.
- Point your left toe outward at an angle and turn your right toe forward.
- Raise your arms so that your palms are facing downward and parallel to the floor. Lean forward and bring your arm and body forward by hinging at the right hip.
- Place your hand on the floor, a yoga block, or your leg.
- Raise your left arm in the direction of the ceiling.
- Looking upward, forward, or down.
- Take a minute or so to maintain this stance.

- Then ensure that you repeat on the other side.

SPHINX YOGA POSE:

Your buttocks and spine are strengthened by this mild backbend. It elongates your stomach, shoulders, and chest.

It could also aid with stress relief.

This pose can help to strengthen muscles such as the glutamal erector spinae muscles major pectoralis, trapezius, and latissimus dorsi.

The guide to doing this yoga is as follows:

- Stretch your legs out behind you while lying on your stomach.
- Use the muscles in your lower back, buttocks, and thighs.
- Keeping your elbows under your shoulders, rest your forearms on the ground with your palms facing down.

- Elevate your head and upper body gradually.
- Lower abdominal muscles should be softly tightened and elevated to assist with back support.
- Make sure you are lifting through your spine and out through the top of your head, not drooping into your lower back.
- Relax in this while keeping a straight line of sight.

COBRA YOGA POSE:

Your shoulders, chest, and belly are all stretched out with this mild backbend pose. This position may help relieve sciatica and strengthen your spine.

In addition, it could aid in reducing the weariness and tension that sometimes accompany back discomfort.

The muscles to stretch are the triceps serratus anterior, gluteus maximus, deltoids, and hamstrings.

The following are the steps to take to do the yoga:

- With your hands behind your shoulders and your fingers pointing forward, lie on your stomach.
- Tightly fold your arms over to your chest. Keep your elbows close to your sides.
Raise your head, shoulders, and chest gradually by applying pressure with your hands.
- Partially, halfway, or fully up can be lifted.
Continue to flex your elbows slightly.
- To make the posture more intense, you might tilt your head back.
- Exhale and release back down to your mat.
Lay your arms down by your sides and place your head back.
- To alleviate lower back strain, slowly sway your hips from side to side.

BRIDGE YOGA POSE:

This inversion and backbend have the potential to be both restorative and exciting. In addition to stretching the spine, it may help with headaches and backaches.

This yoga strengthens the muscles of the rectus and transverse abdominis gluteus as well as the leg muscles (erector spinae).

The guide to doing this yoga is as follows:

- With your heels tucked under your sitting bones and your knees bent, lie on your back.
- Place your arms at your sides. As you raise your tailbone, firmly plant your feet and arms on the ground.
- Lift until your thighs are in line with the floor.
- Keep your arms in their current position, bringing your palms

together with your fingers interlaced behind your hips, or resting your hands beneath your hips for stability.

- Take a minute or so to maintain this stance.
- Release by lowering your spine, vertebra by vertebra, gradually back to the ground.
- Bring both of your knees down.
- Inhale deeply while in this position and relax.

HALF LORD OF THE FISHES YOGA POSE:

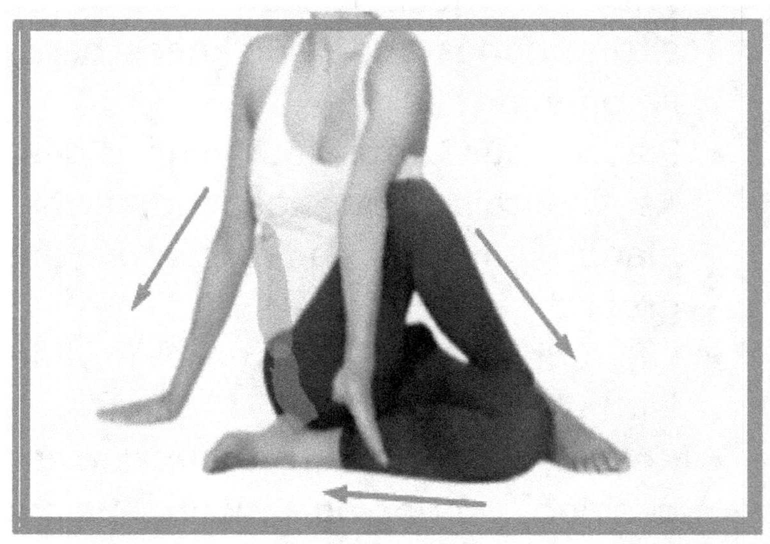

This twisting posture helps to strengthen the muscles like the rhomboids, serratus anterior, erector spinal, pectoralis major, and psoas. It also stretches the muscles in your neck, shoulders, and hips. This pose can assist reduce tiredness and stimulate your internal organs.

The guide to doing this yoga is as follows:

- Bring your right foot in close to your body while seated.
- Place your left foot outside your body.
  Stretch your back and turn your torso to the left.
- For support, place your left hand on the ground behind you.
- Wrap your elbow over your left knee or extend your right upper arm outside of your left leg.
- To make your spine twist more deeply, try to maintain a square hip position.

- Look over your left or right shoulder.
- Take a minute or so to maintain this stance.
- Continue on the opposite side.

TWO-KNEE SPINAL TWIST POSE:

This yoga stretches your neck, upper back, and spine, this rejuvenating twist can help ease pain and stiffness in your hips and back. The muscles employed in this posture include the rectus abdominis, trapezius pectoralis major, and erector spinae.

The guide to doing this yoga is as follows:

- With your arms out to the sides and your knees pulled against your chest, lie on your back.
- Keeping your knees as close together as possible, slowly drop your legs to the left.
- A pillow can be positioned in between or beneath both of your

knees.

You can apply a little pressure on your knees with your left hand.

- You can tilt your neck to one side or keep it straight.
- In this posture, concentrate on taking deep breaths.
- For at least thirty seconds, maintain this position.
- On the other side, repeat.

CHILD'S YOGA POSE:

This yoga helps strengthen the neck and back to feel more relaxed and released as you perform this simple forward fold. Your back is elongated and strained.

In addition, Child's Pose strengthens the ankles, thighs, and hips. This stance may be used to reduce weariness and tension.

The guide to doing this yoga is as follows:

- With your knees together, take a seat back on your heels.

- For support, place a blanket or bolster behind your forehead, chest, or thighs.
- Walk your hands in front of you while bending forward.
- Lay your forehead down lightly on the ground.
- With your palms facing up, hold your arms out in front of you or bring them close to your body.
- As your upper body drops heavily onto your knees, concentrate on releasing tension in your back.
- Hold this position for a maximum of five minutes.

CHAPTER 6: YOGA POSES FOR IMPROVING STRENGTH, BALANCE, MOBILITY AND TO PREVENT INJURY

By strengthening and stabilizing joints even more, these extra yoga poses offer a complete method of promoting joint health.

To prevent strain or injury, always perform these postures attentively and make sure you maintain good alignment and form.

The following are the various yoga poses and how to do them:

THE CAMEL POSE YOGA:

This is a strengthening exercise that strengthens the back, shoulders, and thighs. It also stretches the front of the body, such as the chest, abdomen, and hip flexors.

The following are the steps to begin the pose:

- To perform it, kneel on the floor with your knees hip-width apart.
- Place your hands on your lower back with your fingers pointing down.
- Press your hips forward and lean back, lifting your chest and reaching for your heels with your hands.
- Hold for 30 to 60 seconds, exhaling deeply.

GARUDASANA OR EAGLE YOGA POSE:

This yoga builds strength in the legs, ankles, and core. It stretches the upper back, hips, shoulders, and also. enhances focus and equilibrium.

How to accomplish this pose:

- Place your feet together while standing.
  Lift your right foot and cross it over

your left thigh while bending your knees slightly.

- If at all feasible, place your right foot behind your left calf.
- Bring your hands together and cross your left arm across your right at the elbows.
- After 30 to 60 seconds of holding, switch sides.

DANNCER YOGA POSE:

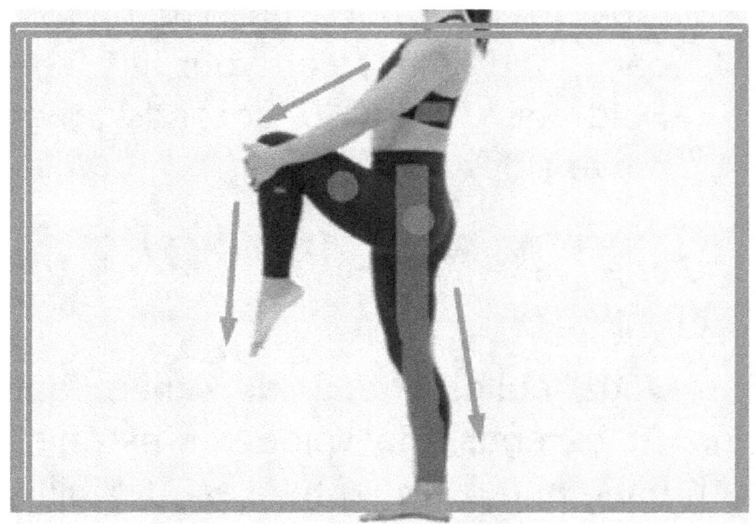

The dancer Pose, also known as Natarajasana helps to build up the ankle joints, legs, and core. It also stretches the quadriceps, shoulders, and hip flexors. It enhances balance and focus.

 The guide to doing this yoga is as follows:

- Start the posse by standing with your feet together, shifting your weight to your left foot, bending your right knee, and bringing your right heel towards your buttocks.
- You then extend your left arm forward, lift your right leg up and back, and balance on your left leg.
- Hold for 30 to 60 seconds, then move sides.

TRIANGLE POSE IN ROTATION (PARIVRTTA TRIKONASANA):

This yoga builds the ankle, knee, and legs. It extends the spine, hamstrings, and hips and also enhances flexibility and balance.

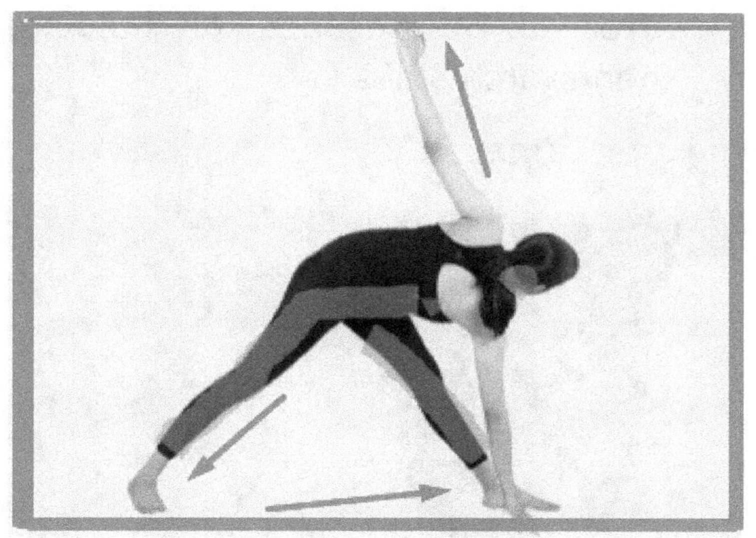

The guide to doing this yoga is as follows:

- Your feet should be placed around 3-4 feet apart.
- Rotate your left foot slightly in and your right foot out 90°.
- With your left hand on the ground or a block outside of your right foot, extend your arms to the sides, then rotate your body to the right.
- Lift your right arm and raise it toward the ceiling while you gaze up at your right hand.

- After 30-60 seconds of holding, then switch sides.

BOAT YOGA POSE:

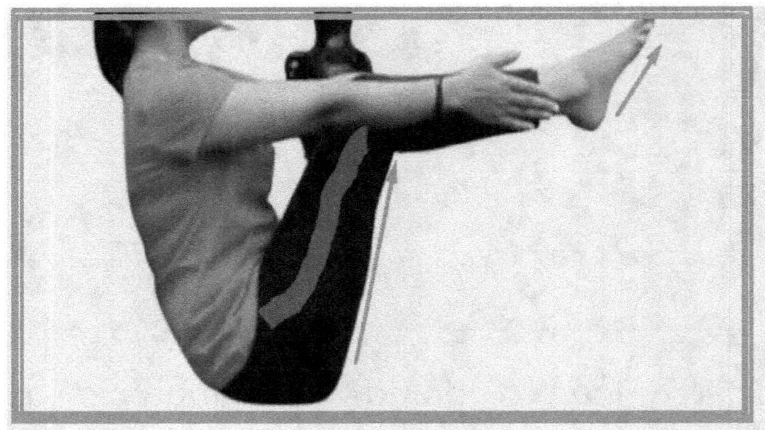

This yoga strengthens the spine, hip flexors, and abdominal muscles. It also increases balance and core stability.

How to do it:

- Sit on the mat with your feet flat and your knees bent.
- Lean back slightly to lift your feet off the floor and balance on your sit bones.
- Stretch your legs straight out in a V-shape with your body.

- Stretch your arms forward, parallel to the floor.
- Hold for 30-60 seconds while taking deep breaths.

Finally, ensure that you pay attention to your body before and when you start each of these yogic poses

If you have any health problems take a break and consult your doctor and if there is any of the yoga you can not do please skip and start with the simple ones.